SPEAK WITH CONFIDENCE: EVEN WITH DENTURES

Training Your Speech Muscles to Attract Clear Communication

Brenda C. Smith

ABOUT THE AUTHOR

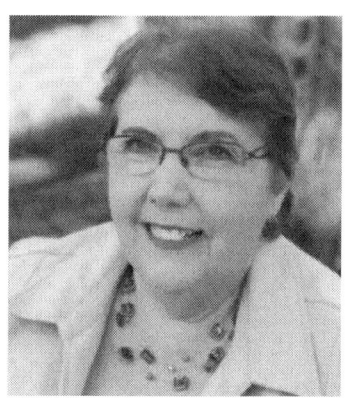

BRENDA C. SMITH, BA, B.ED, A.T.C.L, OCT

Brenda has written several books relating to education and communication throughout her career as a teacher, professor, coach, theatre director, and performer in film, TV, and stage. She has helped thousands of students, professionals, and leaders over 40 years to discover their best voice to speak live or on mic to possess energy and connection to their audiences.

As the Founder of **Voice Power Training Services** she offers online courses and private coaching to corporations, executives, and professional presenters.

"As a speech and drama coach, I'm on your side helping you improve the sound of your voice and your presentation style so you will confidently connect with your listeners."

TABLE OF CONTENTS

Note: *Before doing any of these exercises, always check with a medical professional (ENT Doctor, Speech & Language Pathologist, or Dentist) for any speech disorders, or medical concerns.*

INTRODUCTION

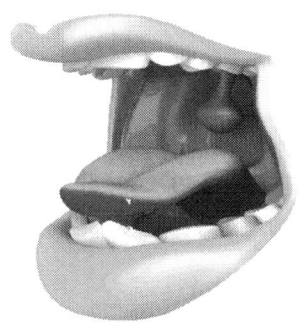

This speech articulation **workout book** is written especially for you if want your message to be understood clearly.

I was personally drawn to writing this book from coaching clients who had new dentures or dental surgery. They suffered from anxiety over not getting their speech quite right, not wanting to socialize or to speak to anyone. It came to focus for me when even more questions came up about this concern during my Voice Power

Workshops, Mastery Online Courses, and at my "Breathe...Just Steps to Breathtaking Speeches" book signing events.

Finally, when my research revealed that this was a major issue globally with most denture wearers, I set to up these articulation exercises to target your speech muscle remedy.

When we are faced with speech challenges or fears, the cause is often inadequate breathing or lazy speech habits. If you've been asked to repeat yourself, accused of mumbling, or now wear dentures; then this is a wake-up call to **work-out** your speech muscles!

The book is organized with each chapter focussing on a primary speech articulator (muscle): jaw, lips, palate, tongue, and teeth, as your speech-muscle team. The chapters begin with a description as to **"What it is,"** so you get to know your speech muscles.

Next**, "How it is Helpful to Speech"** gives you a full explanation as to why articulation involves practice to a specific placement to achieve your end goal of clear communication.

*Note: /b/ -Any letters within slanted lines indicate for you to say the **sound** of the letter; not the name of the letter.*

Under **"How to do the Exercises,"** you can complete key exercises in only 10 minutes and also cherish a **"Favourite Tongue Twister."**

The final section of **"Action Notes"** gives you the exact next steps to do, and a **"Weekly Tracking Calendar,"** to document your progress.

Denture wearers are guided throughout the book on re-training your speech muscles around this new object. I want to support you. Here are the easy tools to prevent your fears and to align everything into a crisp powerful sound.

I'm delighted to lead you through the exercises to transform your speech fears into being confident speakers.

Take the following **"Articulation Checklist Assessment"** before you begin.

ARTICULATION CHECKLIST ASSESSMENT

S peech Muscles consist of your mouth, jaw, lips, tongue, teeth, and palate. This checklist will help you discover your most challenging speech sounds.

Read aloud each item listed below.

Check off the ones MOST DIFFICULT for you to say:

Tongue:

- ❏ Ta-Da; Ta-Da; Tatter, Dad, Dull, Dark Dock
- ❏ Na–No; Need, Nod, Night, Knit
- ❏ La-La-la-la; Lather, Lilly, Low, Lull,
- ❏ Clock, Tuck, Gutter, dock, Key, Care

Lips:

- ☐ Bob, Bam, Pop, Pep, Mummy, Pup, Broom
- ☐ Prep, Brisk, Pepper, Bread, Beast, Beep, Apple

Teeth:

- ☐ This, They, Then, Theatre, Myth
- ☑ Thrift, Thirty-three, Thousands

Jaw:

- ☐ Wow, Wait, Wonder, Which, What, Where, Why
- ☐ Yes, Yawn, Allan, Ouch, Awe

Sibilant Sounds:

- ☐ Sister, Snake, Sauces, Sally, Soccer
- ☑ Miss, Blister, Missiles, Story, Sorry
- ☑ Shout, Shore, Shampoo, Share, Show, Shush

Fricative Sounds:

- ☐ Fa, Fa, Fa; Fluffy, Furry, Four, Fifty, Flap

- ❏ Victory, Valour, Have, Half, Harvey, Fat-Vat
- ❏ Zoo, Zap, Zipper, Puzzle, Booze, Zero

R- sounds:

- ❏ Round, Rap, Roar, Rate, Rather, River, Roger
- ❏ Trapper, Drawer, Saran Wrap, War, Ringer

How did you do on this checklist? You will find all these sounds are addressed in the following chapters. If you find it's only one sound that is causing you challenges, then go directly to that chapter to try those exercises. Get ready to overcome your fear of speaking after dentures.

Chapter 1

MOBILIZE YOUR MOUTH

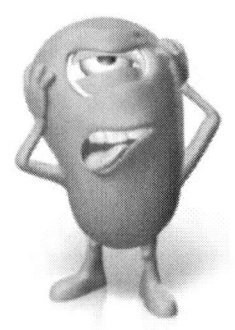

What is it?

Articulation involves the use of the mouth, lips, teeth, palate, tongue, and jaw to produce clear pronunciation and better communication. Always exaggerate their movement while doing an exercise for the best results.

With Dentures you must retrain the muscle memory of your articulators to work around the denture. You are reintroducing where your tongue and other articulators need to land. It will be a new texture, space, and location that the tongue will feel with your denture.

Take your time as you practice for about 10 minutes each day around the dentures. As you limber up, you'll gradually notice how your tongue gets better at muscle memory of where to go, so you are no longer sputtering nonsense.

Why it's Helpful for Speech?

Tight or tense muscles espe-cially in your face, neck, and shoulders will affect your voice (larynx) for pitch levels and your speech muscles for clarity. Imagine if you forgot to oil up your bike and every-

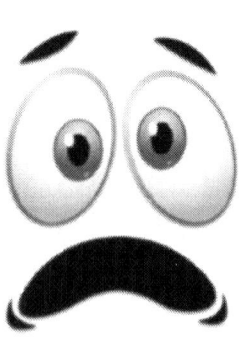

thing became too tight and unmovable. The pur-pose of warming up your speech muscles is to make your speech more fluid and ready to go.

How to do the Exercises:

WARM-UP TO LOOSEN SPEECH MUSCLES

Did you know that every muscle in your body affects your speech? Look at yourself in a mirror while doing your exercises, and have fun with them, so you can enjoy the time working out. Perform the exercises while wearing your dentures. Stop if it hurts and try again when you're ready. It's the daily little steps that will lead to your final puzzle being solved.

Wiggle your Face and Make *Funny Faces*:

1. Scrunch your face tightly then loosen it up. (five times)

2. Make an UGLY face, then a FUNNY face. (five times)

3. Massage your cheeks gently with your fingers for 20 seconds.

4. Wiggle your jaw loosely with the aide of your hand.

5. Open your mouth widely with a BIG SLOW YAWN.

6. Bring your shoulders up to meet your ears then down again. (five times).

7. Look left and right slowly to loosen neck muscles.

8. Move your mouth as you mime chewing gum.

Favourite Tongue Twister: *Gobble, gobble, gobbling gobs*

Action Notes:

I hope you had fun doing the "Wiggle Your Face Exercises", or at least a little chuckle.

● Include your warm-up exercises through-out the day so you become familiar with them; and take a deep breath using your diaphragm to relax yourself before exercising.

● Download here: **"Weekly Tracking Calendar"** to fill in your practice times, exercises, and any notes to track your progress. Or, simply use your phone calendar, or a printed calendar to keep your speech work-out updated.

CHAPTER 2

JUGGLE YOUR JAW

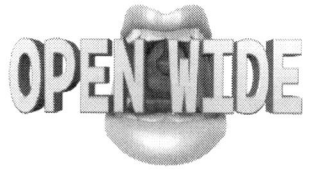

What is it?

The JAW consists of two parts:

1. The **mandible**, or lower jawbone, forms the lower part of the **skull**.

2. The **maxilla**, or upper jaw, forms the **mouth** structure.

Movement of the lower jaw opens and closes the **mouth** and allows for the chewing of food. The lower set of **teeth** in the mouth is rooted in the lower jaw. The upper teeth are attached to the skull.

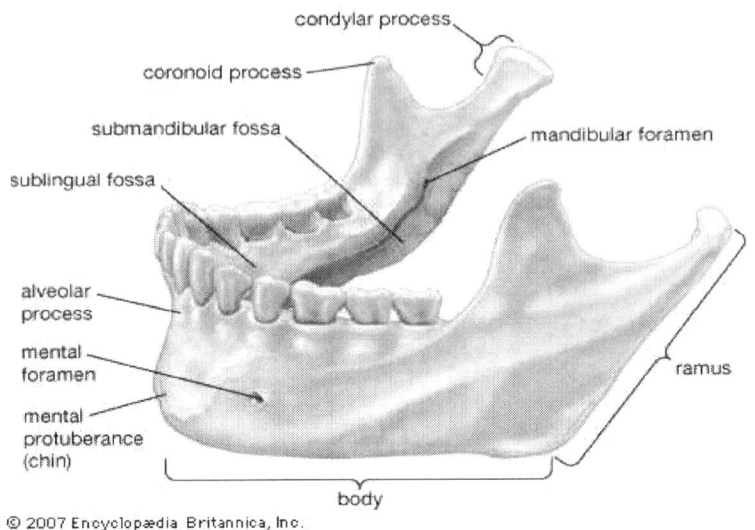

condylar process

coronoid process

submandibular fossa

mandibular foramen

sublingual fossa

alveolar process

mental foramen

mental protuberance (chin)

ramus

body

© 2007 Encyclopædia Britannica, Inc.

Why it's Helpful for Speech?

It is important for Speech because it works as a team player in getting your sound out of your mouth so you can be heard clearly. Loosening your jaw will help to focus your mind on speaking with clear articulation.

Two joints and several jaw muscles, ligaments, and the mandible jawbone make it possible to open and close the mouth. They work together when you chew, speak, or swallow. Located on each side of the head, they work together to make many different movements, including a combination of rotating and gliding actions used when chewing and speaking.

How to do the Exercises:

1. Drop jaw lazily and allow the mouth to fall open.

2. Move the jaw from side to side gently with your hand.

3. Move the jaw around in a circle. Say, **"jaw"** (five times)

4. Say **"ouch"** with wide open mouth on /**ou**/ (five times).

5. Repeat "gabble" with mouth wide on /**a**/ (five times).

6. Say, **"WOW"** five times stretching your open jaw.

7. Take a huge **YAWN** of air and hold for 4 seconds.

8. Exaggerate a wide mouth for the stressed vowels in this sentence: "I watched the white whale from my yacht." (two times)

Favourite Tongue Twister:

A wagon wobbled widely and wildly.

Action Notes:

Add Warm-ups before the speech exercises

- Say, "Jaw" throughout the day dropping your jaw as you say it.

CHAPTER 3

LUBRICATE YOUR LIPS

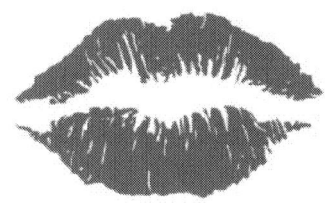

What is it?

Bilabial refers to your two lips, upper and lower, which come together to make a sound. When your lips smack together, they make a popping sound on the consonants /b/ and /p/ and /m/.

The /W/ sound is made by **rounded** lips: as in "WE."

A **Voiceless** label is given for the sound for /p/, because there is a puff of air that accompanies it; such as in the word, "POP"

A **Voiced** sound is given for the /b/ sound which comes directly from your vocal folds without the puff of air; as in "BOB"

Why it's helpful for speech?

If you have lazy lips the accuracy of those **consonant sounds** will be lost, and your speech will not be understood. The lips are also useful in the formation of **vowel sounds,** a, e, i, o, u as they can change shape, for example, the long vowel "o" by rounding the lips. Or, they can open and stretch into a smile shape, for example, to make sound of "e."

Consonants give the edge to your words, while vowels give the fullness of tone to your words. Look in the mirror to see if your lips are moving when you do these exercises. **Avoid speaking behind your teeth, or denture teeth, without any lip movement as this will prevent your listeners from hearing your sound.**

So, let's exercise moving those lips of yours!

How to do the Exercises:

- Place the palm of your hand in front of your mouth:
  - ○ **Say**, "POP" three times to feel the puff of air on your hand as you say and hear it (voiceless)
  - ○ **Say,** "BOB" three times where you don't feel air on your hand, you just hear it (voiced)

1. **"Smile" and "Kiss"** mid-air five times. This exercise will make your lips more flexible.

2. **Repeat**: "A Big Black Bug Bit a Big Black Bear." (three times). This will get your upper lip to be more flexible, so it is not stiff.

3. **Say** these **"M"** words: Mom, Mommy, many, miles, minimal, mumble, moan, memory, ambush, mammoth

4. **Say**, "**oo-ee**" with round lips and wide-open lips. (five times).

5. **Repeat:** "Bobby mumbled that Mommy Bear had many miles to make before meeting Poppa Bear." (three times).

With dentures your lips may have to re-adjust as to where your teeth are positioned in relation to your mouth size, shape, or gum line.

Avoid clicking sounds of your dentures while speaking by slowing down with your exercises, speaking, and noticing which words are causing the clicking sounds.

Favourite Tongue Twister:

Peter Piper picked a peck of pickled peppers.

Action Notes:

● See your dentist if your dentures come loose when you're talking, laughing, or eating. They may not fit properly in your mouth. Your gum and bones change with age; and your gum recedes after your teeth have been removed for your new dentures.

- Repeat often these two tongue twisters from this chapter:
  - A big black bug bit a big black bear
  - Peter Piper picked a peck of pickled peppers

Chapter 4

TRIGGER YOUR TONGUE

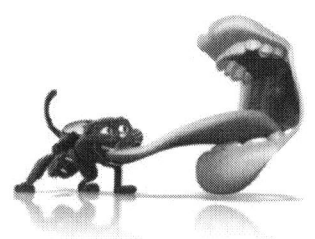

What is it?

Your tongue is the strongest muscle. It consists of the tongue tip, the tongue blade (wide flat mid section) and the back of the tongue. It's the major speech articulator interacting with the teeth, gum, lips, palate, and jaw to create many specific sounds.

Why it's Helpful for Speech?

The Tongue Tip taps behind your front teeth on your upper gum (alveolar ridge) to create the /t/ (voiceless) sound as in the word "**tap**," and the /d/ (voiced) sound, as in "**Dad**."

Your /N/ sound as in "**N**o" has the tongue placed there too. You will have more exercises for the "**n**" in Chapter 6.

However, the placement of tongue for hard guttural sounds /g/, /k/, and **hard** /c/ <u>arches the tongue in the back of your mouth</u>: as in these words: **G**o, **K**ey, **C**ook.

The placement of your tongue for /L/ sound is a tongue-tip flip on upper palate just behind the upper teeth, for example, as in saying the word "**lily.**"

Placement of tongue for the **"th"** sound is between the upper and lower teeth which will be covered under the Teeth Chapter 5.

How to do the Exercises:

1. Warm-up your tongue first:

    a. Stick your tongue out of your mouth and circle it around the outside of your mouth and lips. Go in both directions right (clockwise) three times, and then left (anti-clockwise), three times.

b. Move your tongue inside your mouth to left cheek then to right cheek while pushing your cheeks out. (three times).

c. Point the tip of your tongue upward just behind your front teeth; then drag the tip across the roof of your mouth, the hard palate, to the back as far as the soft palate.

d. Touch your tongue onto your lower teeth and flip it under while pushing the rest of your tongue (blade) outward through your teeth and mouth.

2. **Repeat:** "Red Leather, Yellow Leather" (five times). This gives your tongue a great workout on the /L/ and the /TH/.

3. **Repeat the sounds of** Ta-Da, Ta-Da, Ta-Da (three times).

Favourite Tongue Twister:

Lillory, lollory, lallory

Action Notes:

- Read from a book for 10 minutes

CHAPTER 5

TARGET YOUR TEETH

What is it?

Dentures are now replacing your upper and lower teeth; so, the tongue must manoeuvre around and between the teeth; and touch your gum ridge, and palate freely.

Why it's Helpful for Speech?

Your **tongue and teeth are Partners** in creating accurate speech for the sounds of "**th**." For this sound, the placement of your the Tongue **TIP** must come slightly out of your mouth between your top and bottom teeth. Allow for air to pass out. These 'th" words are part of the "**Fricative**" group of speech sounds

- For a **voiceless** (**soft**) "**th**" you should feel more air (breath) escape - e.g. *MYTH*

- For a **voiced** (hard) 'th" you should hear sound coming from the vocal folds with no puff of air -e.g. *THEY*

How to do the Exercises:

A. Voiceless "th" is at the <u>initial, mid, or final</u> part of the word.

1. Look in the mirror to determine if your tongue tip is seen **between your teeth** when you pronounce the "**th**:"

- *thin - something - bath*;

- *thought - birthday - truth*;

- third - filthy - health;

2. Read aloud these sentences:

1. It's **thin**.

2. He **thought** about the war.

3. It's a lovely **thimble**.

4. He gave his dog a **bath**.

C. **Voiced "th"** - is also at the <u>initial, mid, or final</u> part of the word. The placement is exactly like the previous "th" except that it is voiced, heard from your larynx.

1. **Repeat these words:**

   - **th**e - fa**th**er - smoo**th**

   - **th**ere - wea**th**er - brea**th**e;

   - **th**us, - ei**th**er - tee**th**

2. **Read aloud these sentences:**

   1. **They** began early.

   2. The child is **teething**

   3. It's a very **worthy** cause.

Contrast saying the **"th"** words spoken **between** your teeth **with** those **"t" and "d"** words that **touch** the upper gum ridge (alveolar ridge) behind the upper front teeth.

1. **"They** began early." versus "The **Day** began early."

2. "He threw the **leather** away." versus "He threw the **letter** away."

3. "The child is **teething,**" with "The child is **teasing.**"

4. "You'll see her **mother**;" with "You'll see her **mutter.**"

Favourite Tongue Twister:

Thirty thousand thoughtless thieves

Action Notes:

Wow! You're half-way through your journey. Great work! Keep tracking your progress on your calendar.

Let's see how you are progressing with getting the edge, beginning, and ends, of each the words.

● **Read this passage** from Shakespeare's "Hamlet"

"Speak the speech, I pray you, as I pronounced it to you, trippingly on the tongue. But if you mouth it, as many of your players do, I had as life the town crier spoke my lines,"

— William Shakespeare,

Hamlet (3.2. 1-4)

CHAPTER 6

PUMP YOUR SOFT PALATE

What is it?

The upper part of your mouth, often called the roof of your mouth is the palate. It consists of two parts: an upper hard palate from the front of mouth to the mid-section; and the soft palate section at the back of your mouth.

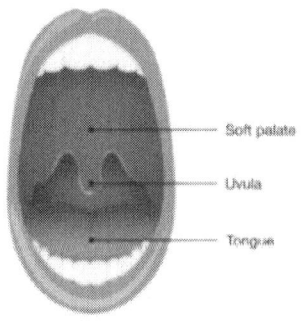

Upper Airway Anatomy Front View

Soft palate

Uvula

Tongue

This **soft palate**, or **velum**, contains muscles to make it move up or down. The attached small hanging tissue in the centre of the soft palate is called the **uvula**. The action of the soft palate rises to close off the passage to your nose so your sound will exit the mouth. It also lowers itself to block off the mouth entrance at the throat or pharynx so your nasal sound will exit the nose. All sounds except for *m, n, and ng* will exit the mouth.

Why it's helpful for speech?

M, N, NG:

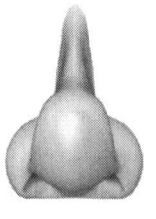

A nasal tone is produced on the sounds of /m/, /n/, and /ng/ because the breath passes through the **nasal** cavity (nose) instead of the **oral** cavity (the mouth).

The soft palate, or velum, at the back of your mouth rises to block the breath from escaping via the mouth.

If you have a **lazy soft palate,** then you may have too nasal a tone because your vowel sounds are exiting the nose instead of the mouth.

To avoid nasality of tone (except *m, n, ng*) exercise your **soft palate**.

How to do the Exercises:

RAISE AND LOWER YOUR VELUM AT THE BACK OF YOUR THROAT:

Be aware of these tongue and soft palate placements before you start the exercise below. First, while speaking with /n/, and /ng/ sounds, your tongue arches up in the back of your throat while your velum rises to block these sounds from exiting the mouth. Instead, it escapes through your nasal passage to create a nasal tone or twang sound.

Second, say /awe/ and notice that your jaw will drop to emit sounds from your wide mouth opening and the tongue lies low in your mouth. There is no longer any nasal tone.

Exercises:

1. **Say**, /ung/ (nasal) as in "sung" (five times); then **say** /awe/ (mouth). (five times)

2. **Repeat together**: 'ung-aw.' (five times)

3. **Repeat:** "sing" (three times); then say "law" (no nasal). (three times)

4. **Say**, "The sun rises slowly awakening the day." (three times)

5. **Repeat** these words: tongue, singer, belonging, think, finger, anxious, handkerchief. (two times)

Favourite Tongue Twister:

Ninety-nine Nuns hummed hymns until noon.

Action Notes:

Teach your tongue to become accustomed to your new dentures.

- Exercise your tongue going up in the back of your throat so the velum is raised to make it more active on the /ng/ sounds

- Stretch your mouth wide open with a big yawn as a warm-up to these exercises

- Repeat the exercise that is giving you the most challenge.

CHAPTER 7

SIZZLE YOUR SIBILANTS

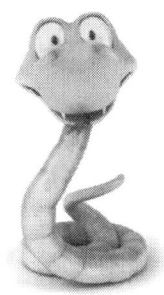

What is it?

Sibilant sounds are the **"s"** (voiceless) and **"z"** (voiced) sounds. They are made by forcing air through a small passage between the front of the tongue and the tooth ridge. The lips are slightly spread open during this sound.

For similar sounds "sh" (voiceless) and "zh" (voiced) the mid section of your tongue is arching

31

up toward the back of the palate or roof of your mouth. A slight rounding of the lips happens as sound escapes around the tongue.

Why it's Helpful for Speech?

If you tongue position is in the wrong position or lazy your speech sounds may exaggerate the whistle sound too much, or it may sound sloppy and unclear, or sound as if there is a lisp.

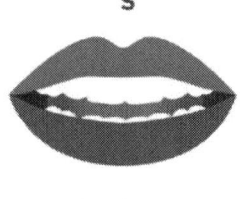

s

swim | same

The **"s"** makes a long high pitch hissing sound, e.g. "**S**ue." as the air escapes. The soft letter "c" makes the same /s/ sound, e.g. **C**ity

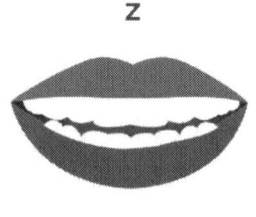

z

zoo | zipper

The **"z"** makes a short hiss that is voiced, e.g. "zoo."

SH

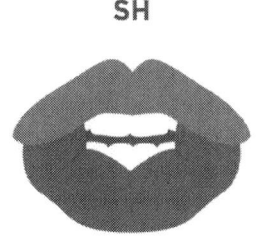

she | fish

The "**sh**" has the tongue arched but more relaxed, e.g. "**ships**"

The "zh" sound is voiced, e.g. "chips"

There are numerous other spellings that sound "sh" or "zh:"- e.g. "ch," "tu," "tion," "su" ... and more.

- church, Chicago, nature, ocean, station, watch, chair

How to do the Exercises:

"s" – "z":

1. **Alternate** saying /**ss zz ss zz**/ maintaining the same articulation placement. (two times)

2. **Repeat**: *yes, smile, cycle, house, loose, class, discuss, collapse.* (two times)

3. **Repeat**: *buzz, frozen, easy, his, these, goes, zone, music, reason.* (two times)

"SH" – "ZH":

1. **Repeat**: "ssh!", *should, brush, she, wish, permission, appreciate, cautious, negotiate.* (two times)

2. **Repeat**: *church, picture, scratch, fortune, machine, measure, culture, porch. (*two times)

3. **Say:** The snake hisses slowly slithering silently up the slippery slope.

Say the following sentences of voiceless and voiced:

1. They **sipped** tea slowly.   - They **zipped** through traffic.

2. The **prices** are excellent. - The **prizes** are excellent.

3. She took my **share**.   - She took my **chair**.

Favourite Tongue Twister:

Sister Sue sews shirts, shorts, shoulder straps for soldiers.

Action Notes:

- These are tricky ones; but look how far you've come so you deserve to give yourself a pat on the back.

- Take three diaphragmatic breaths before doing your exercises, so you don't get anxious. You can pause any time and breathe again to calm yourself.

- Discover which one of the sibilant exercises above is the most difficult for you. Then focus on repeating only that one.

CHAPTER 8

FIX YOUR FRICATIVES

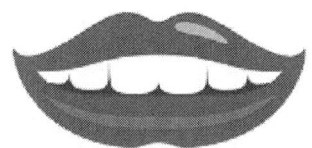

F,V

What is it?

Fix Your Fricatives: /f/, /v/ Placement:

The lower lip moves up to touch the upper teeth as the air streams out with a slight hissing noise (friction). The upper lip remains still, no rounding, as the inside lower lip slightly touches the edges of the upper teeth.

Why it's Helpful for Speech?

The **articulation** of both /f/ **voiceless**, and /v/ **voiced** are the same. You should clearly see your two front teeth in the mirror. Also, squeeze the bottom lip and upper teeth together and force air out of the mouth the whole time.

The **voiced** /v/ holds the air flow continuously to create the friction you will feel in the mouth. Plus, you will hear the **voicing produced at the larynx**.

Look in the mirror to be sure they look the same as you **compare /f/ and /v/** while saying these word pairs:

- Lea**f** - Lea**v**e
- **F**airy - **V**ery
- Sa**f**er – Sa**v**er
- **F**ail – **V**eil

You should be able to go easily between the two to hear a difference so your listener will know the correct word right away.

Other spellings have the fricative sounds: "ph" and "gh" as in "phone" and "laugh."

How to do the EXERCISES:

1. **Voiceless "f"** - Practise saying the following:

   a. Fan, leaf, effort, off, enough, laugh, cough, rough, photograph, alphabet, sphere

   b. They laughed at the awful photograph of Fred falling off a fence.

2. **Voiced "v"** – Practise saying the following to make the formation the same **as /f/:**

   a. Van, voice, leave, develop, every, carve, of-(voiced "f")

   b. We voted in favour of giving everyone five days of vacation.

3. **Practise both /f/ and /v/ sentences.** *Vowels are lengthened before a final /v/*

   a. I'd like a **view**.   - I'd like a **few**.

   b. Do you want to **have** an apple? - Do you want **half** an apple?

Favourite Tongue Twister:

Fickle frittering, frittering fickle

Action Notes:

- Repeat any difficult /v/ exercises and add in the /w/ sound with rounded lips for better accuracy.

- For example, say, "That's a nice vine;" then say, "That's a nice wine."

- Say, "I think it's a verse," and "I think it's worse."

- Smile, and have fun with the exercises.

- Practise speaking socially, and on the phone; you can do this!

Chapter 9

RALLY YOUR "R'S"

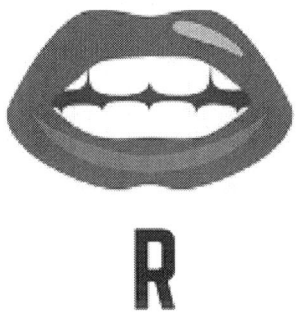

What is it?

Placement of your tongue is at mid to back of throat arched up to the palate while your lips are rounded. Air flows over the center of the tongue without the tongue tip touching any part of palate (roof of mouth). Make your lips round first then say "errrrr."

A **Blended R sound** consists of a **Consonant + /r/'** such as, initial sounds: /tr/, /br/, /cr/, /dr/, /fr/, etc for all consonants. You combine the two sounds into one sound, e.g. **br**eed, **cr**ayon, **dr**ill, **fr**og,

Middle and Final sounds with vowel will take **Vowel sound combined with /r/,** e.g. ca**r**, dee**r**, si**r**, fo**r**, fu**r**.

OR

ER

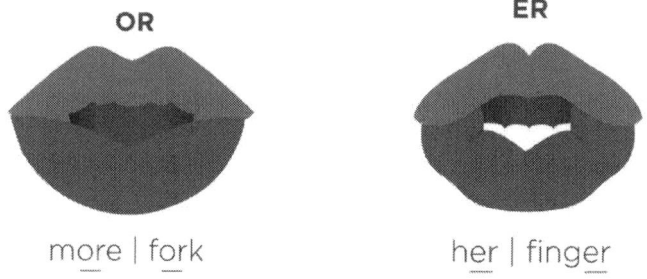

more | fork   her | finger

Why it's Helpful for Speech?

How to do the Exercises:
Practice saying words and sentences:

1. A**r**ound, **r**ed, a**rr**ive, **r**ock, **r**ip, **r**ide, **r**oad, **tr**ain, hu**rr**y, **cr**owd, **thr**ow, **rh**ythm, **tr**ue, **tr**y, ze**r**o, **str**ing, **pr**ay

2. The **pr**ofessor **tr**avelled **thr**ough the **cr**owd as he hu**rr**ied to a**rr**ive befo**r**e it sta**r**ted to **r**ain.

42

3. **Record saying the following** to test yourself with your other pronunciation sounds:

- Would you like **r**oast **l**amb with **r**ice?
- The **shr**ewd manag**er** solved any **pr**oblem by giving coupons for **free** dinn**ers.**
- The **gr**ass is still wet. - *The glass is still wet*
- It's a la**r**ge **r**ing.   - *It's a large wing.*
- Are you going to **fr**y them? - Are you going to **fl**y them?

Favourite Tongue Twister:

Around the rough and rugged rocks the ragged rascals rudely ran.

Action Notes:

- Record yourself reading aloud a paragraph from a book
- Update your tracking calendar

CHAPTER 10

ARTICULATE TO ATTRACT

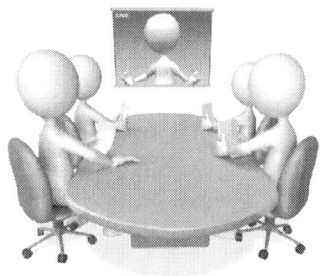

What is it?

S peaking your words distinctly for coher-
ent and fluent expression to achieve
clear communication

Why it's helpful for speech?

Getting the **edge** of your words is **clear** enun-
ciation for your listeners not to be confused as

to which words you're saying. This avoids mumbling with garbled speech, speaking too quickly, and pronouncing unclear speech. For example, if you drop the **end** of the word "fad" and the listener only heard you say, "fa.." Then a listener thinks you might have said, "fat," or "far," or 'fall;" or some other word.

Initial sounds are critical as well. Imagine if you confused these two words: "produce" and "reduce" because you rushed through your articulation of the initial sound of the word. Half your listeners heard "produce" while the other half heard "reduce." This would certainly create chaos if you happened to be speaking to your sales group, or your factory line workers, or your bank manager.

With crystal clear articulation your listeners perk up and pay attention to what your message is.

How to do the Exercises: Repeat each one three times before doing the next one.

Practise these 25 tongue twisters for **clarity not for speed:**

1. The wagon wobbled wildly and widely.
2. Giggle, giggle, giggling girls
3. Kick, kick, kicking cows
4. Gobble, gobble, gobbling gobs
5. Trickle, trickle, trickling streams
6. twinkle, twinkle, twinkling twins
7. Bubble, bubble, bubbling blobs
8. Drizzle, drizzle, drizzling drains
9. Fickle, frittering, frittering fickle
10. Good blood, bad blood
11. Peter Piper picked a peck of pickled peppers.
12. Around the rough and rugged rocks, the ragged rascals rudely ran.
13. Sister Sue sewed shirts, shorts, shoulder straps for soldiers.
14. Sixty-six sick chicks

15. A big black bug bit a big black bear.

16. Rubber buggy baby bumpers

17. Thirty thousand thoughtless thieves

18. Lillory, lollory, lallory

19. Truly rural, rural truly

20. Red leather, yellow leather

21. Satter, setter, sitter

22. Prasp, presp, prisp

23. Smith's crisps

24. Toy boats

25. Speak with the lips, the teeth, the tip of the tongue.

Now it's your turn to choose:

What is YOUR Favourite Tongue Twister?

Action Notes:

- Do a daily warm-up and practise many favourite tongue twisters

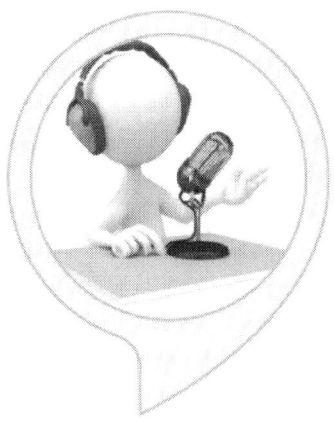

Hey, there's an ALEXA APP of these exercises, that I developed so you can say, "Alexa, OPEN SPEAK CLEARLY WARMUPS." Alexa will give you one daily or whenever you ask for it. She repeats each one randomly saying it three times to guide you through together. If this is something that might help you to warmup your speech muscles, then please use it.

CONCLUSION

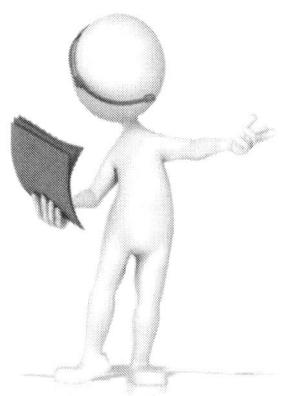

We form and shape our speech or language by our articulators: the lips, teeth, tongue, palate, and jaw. They work in concert with the oral cavity (the mouth), the hard and soft palate (roof of your mouth). Lazy articulators cause incomplete speech clarity and result in a muddied version of the word that you intended to say.

Even a simple ending to a word can be missed by the listener because you, as the speaker, do not enunciate crisply; or you rush through your sentences, or you mumble the words.

When your mouth suddenly has a Denture, then your speech articulators need to be retrained around this new object.

Congratulations for completing this speech-muscle workout! Wear your dentures proudly; everyone now hears you speaking clearly without being aware that you are wearing dentures.

Smile! Your dentures look great and you've retrained you articulators to feel right at home.

"Speak with the lips, the teeth, and the tip of the tongue."

Here's to Keeping Voice Fit!

Appendix

RESOURCES

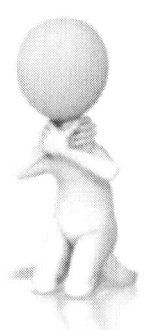

1. Download this Weekly Tracking Calendar: http://bit.ly/2KM1Vlf

2. Download here: "Taking Care of Your Voice" http://bit.ly/2NjqnTu

3. Click this title to play "Speak with Dentures Key Exercises" Video:

4. Here is a summary chart of consonants: From "Breathe...Just Steps to Breathtaking Speeches" —Brenda C. Smith, Chapter 4. p. 72

Voiceless(whispered)	Voiced (spoken)
/p/ as in pit	/b/ as in bit
/t/ as in tent	/d/ as in dent
/f/ as in fat	/v/ as in vat
/s/ as in sit	/z/ as in zit
/th/ as in with	/th/ as in this
/k/ as in cake or kite	/g/ as in gate
/sh/ as in show	/zh/ as measure
/hw/ as in where*	/w/ as in were
	/n/ as in net
	/m/ as in met
*/hw/ is simplified to /w/ in many languages	

5. Check out our websites for online coaching courses and more resources: www.voicepowertraining.com and www.brendacsmith.com

Printed in Great Britain
by Amazon

33417501R00045